TRACE ELEMENTS
IN OBSTETRICS AND GYNECOLOGY

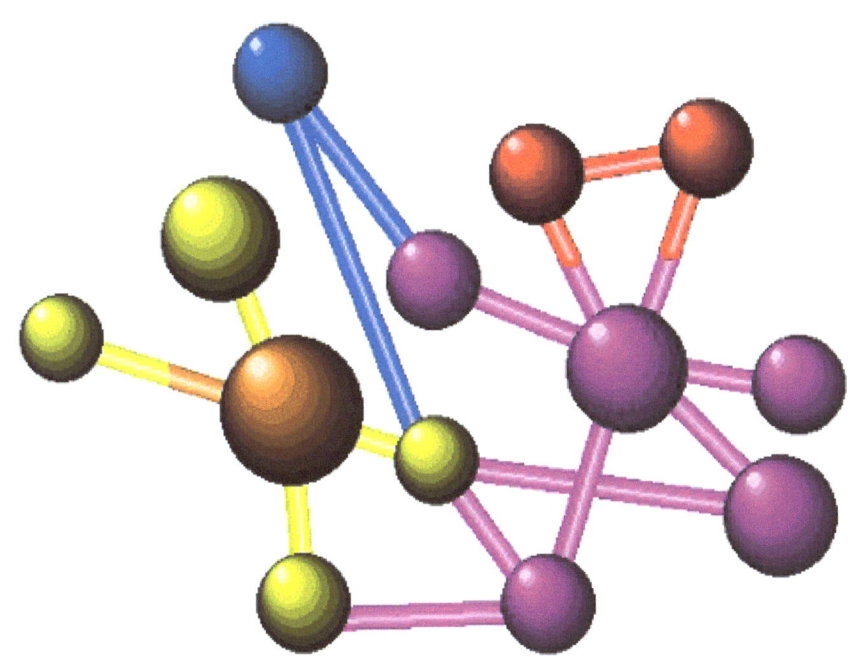

Naira R. Matevosyan, M.D, Ph. D

ISBN: 978-1482393828 / Copyright © 2013 with CreateSpace, Inc.
7290 Investment Dr, North Charleston, SC 29418

CONTENTS

DEFINITON, SIGNIFICANCE, TRACING

Trace element is a chemical element required in *minute quantities* to maintain proper physical functioning. Cobalt (Co), copper (Cu), germanium (Ge), iron (Fe), manganese (Mn), molybdenum (Mo), nickel (Ni), rubidium (Rb), selenium (Se), stibium or antimony (Sb), strontium (Sr), or zinc (Zn) out of the 72 vital trace elements (TE), are presented in very small amounts in biomedical samples (plasma, urine, saliva, cerebro-spinal fluid, full-term placenta, hair, nails, buccal mucosa, semen, biopsy specimens), but these are essential for our optimal development, effective immune defense, metabolic functioning, reproduction, and even pain alleviation. Certain heavy metals, such as arsenic (As), cadmium (Cd), chromium (Cr), lead (Pb), mercury (Hg) or thallium (Ti) are necessary for our metabolism in nearly microscopic amounts; their excess can be toxic.

In *analytical chemistry*, TE are the elements with an average concentration of less than 100 parts per million measured in atomic count or less than 100 micrograms per gram. In *biochemistry*, TE are dietary minerals needed in very minute quantities. In *geochemistry*, TE are chemical elements with concentrations less than 1000 ppm or 0.1% of a rock's composition.

In *life sciences*, TE are measured through sensitive wavelength selection methods combined with *Visible/near infrared atomic absorption spectroscopy* (Vis/NIR), *refractive index* (RI) counts, *Total reflection X-ray fluorescence analysis* (TXRF), *Particle-induced X-ray emission* (PIXE), *Non-flame atomization*, *Nuclear microscopy*, *Voltametry*, and *Chemometrics.* [1-3]

Trace-elemental analysis in clinical samples has received increasing attention in recent years. Consequently, the demands on analytical instrumentation to address the challenges involved in TE measurement in clinical samples have also increased. Historically, *Graphite furnace atomic absorption spectroscopy* (GFAAS) has been the technique of choice in this field, owing to its ability to accurately measure many analytes at trace levels in a range of sample matrices, and in many cases, GFAAS remains the technique of choice. However, relatively long analysis times, limited multi-element capability and complex, analyte dependent sample preparation requirements (the use of chemical modifiers to stabilize target elements during the ashing process or to promote vaporisation in the measuring stage) have led analysts to investigate the potential of *Inductively coupled plasma mass spectrometry* (ICP-MS) for some of their applications.

ICP-MS is an analytical technique used for elemental determinations. Commercially introduced in 1983, the technique has gained general acceptance in multi-profile laboratories. Geochemical labs were early adopters of ICP-MS technology because of its superior detection capabilities, particularly for the GFAAS: (1) higher throughput; (2) the ability to handle both simple and complex matrices with a minimum of matrix interferences due to the high-temperature of the ICP source; and (3) the ability to obtain isotopic information.

Figure 1 shows the schematic representation of an ICP source in an ICP-

MS and fate of the sample:

Here, the ICP source converts the atoms of the elements in the sample to ions. These ions are then separated and detected by the mass spectrometer. Argon gas flows inside the concentric

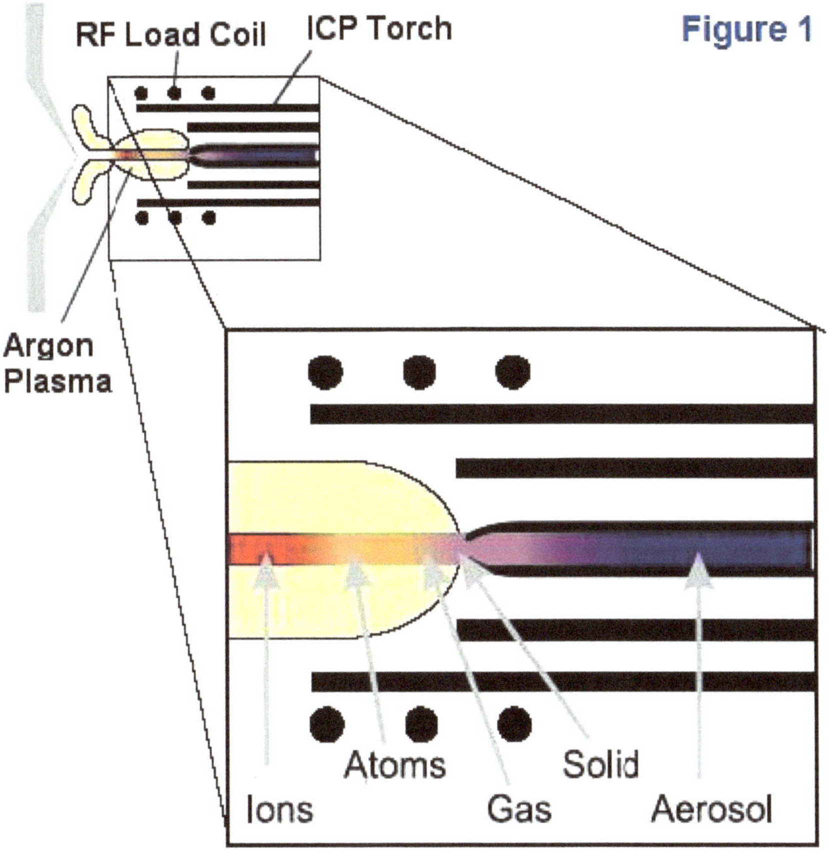

Figure 1

channels of the ICP torch. The radio-frequency load coil is connected to a RF generator. As power is supplied to the load coil from the generator, oscillating electric and magnetic fields are established at the end of the torch. When a spark is applied to the argon flowing through the ICP torch, electrons are stripped off of the argon atoms, forming argon ions. These ions are caught in the oscillating fields and collide with other argon atoms, forming an argon discharge or plasma.

The sample is typically introduced into the ICP plasma as an aerosol, either by aspirating a liquid or dissolved solid sample into a nebulizer or using a laser to directly convert solid samples into an aerosol. Once the sample aerosol is introduced into the ICP torch, it is completely dissolved and the elements in the aerosol are converted first into gaseous atoms and then ionized towards the end of the plasma. [4]

With the advent of collision and reaction cell technology for ICP-MS, the interference problems that previously limited the capability of this technique for measurement of Se in particular (Ar^{2+} interferes with ^{76}Se, ^{78}Se and ^{80}Se) in clinical samples have been largely overcome. Sulfur (S) has long been known to be a useful material in which to measure elements such as Cu, Zn and Se for diagnosis and monitoring of certain diseases and for nutritional studies. It is a complex matrix substance that consists of inorganic salts and a high concentration of protein (approximately 70 g/l), together with a variety of trace substances. [5]

TE will either prefer liquid or solid phase. If compatible with a mineral, it will prefer a solid phase. TE can be substituted for network-forming cations in mineral structures. Minerals do not have to contain trace elements. TE do not have to appear in the mineral's chemical formula. If incompatible with an element, a TE will prefer a liquid phase. The measurement of this ratio is known as the *partition coefficient.*

PARTITION COEFFICIENT AND HENRY'S LAW

A trace element is defined as any element present below ~0.1 wt. %. Units such as *ppm* (parts per million), *ppb* (parts per billion), *ppt* (parts per trillion), and *ppq* (parts per quintillion) are some of the units used to describe the concentrations of TE in a bio-liquid or tissues. Because TE are present in such small quantities, they generally exert minimal control on the state of a system. For example, in silicate systems, TE rarely form mineral phases, and in aqueous systems, they do not form major species.

The distribution of TE within a system is controlled by how it is partitioned among various phases. The partitioning between various phases (mineral and melt phases) occurs in a predictable manner. In addition, a number of TE decay radioactively to another trace-element, allowing the isotopic composition of such daughter elements to be used to constrain the timescales of petrologic processes that fractionate parent/daughter elemental ratios.

The ratio of the concentration of a TE in one phase relative to another phase is called the ***partition coefficient.*** In general, the partition coefficient of an element ***i*** for a given mineral ***j*** is defined to be the ratio of its concentration in the mineral to that in the melt at equilibrium:

$$D^i_j = \frac{C^i_j}{C^i_{Melt}}$$

When $D < 1$, the element is incompatible in the mineral, it is in the melt. When $D > 1$, the element is compatible and stays in the solid. If more than one mineral is crystallizing from a magma, the behavior of the trace element may be described by a bulk distribution coefficient (Di) where

$$\overline{D}_i = \sum_{\varphi} X_{\varphi} D_i^{\varphi}$$

$X\varphi$ is the weight fraction of phase φ, and $Di\varphi$ is the distribution coefficient for component i in phase φ.

For a rock, consisting of several phases j, the bulk partition coefficient is given by the weighted average of the individual partition coefficients for each phase,

$$D_B^i = \sum_j X_j \frac{C_j^i}{C_{Melt}^i}$$

where Xj presents the weight fraction of the j - the phase *in the solids*.

More generally, we can describe TE partitioning as an exchange reaction between the melt and the coexisting mineral. For example, we can describe the partitioning of Ni^{2+} between olivine (ol) and melt as an exchange reaction without the need to specify a melt structure:

$0.5Mg_2SiO_4$ (ol) $+ Ni^{2+}$ (melt) $= 0.5Ni_2SiO_4$ (ol) $+ Mg^{2+}$ (melt)

For non-ideal mixing, the activity coefficients deviate from unity. Two scenarios arise. If both activity coefficients are constant over a wide compositional range (but near infinite dilution of the TE), the TE's behavior in the mineral and melt follows Henry's Law which states that *"at a constant temperature, the amount of a given gas that dissolves in a given type and volume of liquid is directly proportional to the partial pressure of that gas in equilibrium with that liquid."* [6]

In geophysics, a version of Henry's law applies to the solubility of a noble gas in contact with silicate melt. One equation used is

$$C_{melt}/C_{gas} = \exp\left[-\beta(\mu_{melt}^{E} - \mu_{gas}^{E})\right]$$

where:

C = the number concentrations of the solute gas in the melt and gas phases

β = 1/kBT, an inverse temperature scale (BT is the Boltzmann constant)

μE = the excess chemical potentials of the solute gas in the two phases.

In the Henry's Law region, the partition coefficient for a particular TE does not depend on its concentration in the mineral or melt. But if the activity coefficient varies as a function of concentration of the element of interest, then non-Henrian behavior is displayed. This means that the partition coefficient cannot be constant. It is critically important when applying measured partition coefficients to evaluate whether Henry's Law is obeyed.

In clinical studies on biological samples, the partition coefficient of certain TE is important in cancer diagnosis, staging, and prognosis. For example, more than 20 biologically relevant TE distributions in carcinomas of the digestive tract are determined by total reflection X-ray fluorescence analysis (TXRF). The concentration of Ca is found to be virtually constant (0.250 μg per 0.1 mm^3) in normal tissue and in carcinoma of the digestive organs. However, a significant diminution of Cr, Fe and Ni in carcinoma of the stomach, Cr and Co - in carcinoma of the colon, a significant accumulation of potassium (K) in cancerous tissue of the colon, Fe and K - in neoplastic tissue of the rectum are determined for being prognostic. [7]

In animal studies, through the nuclear microscopy, Rutherford backscattering spectrometry and proton induced X-ray emission it is established, that the accurate measurements of Fe and Zn in newly formed atherosclerotic lesions helps with prognosis. Fe concentrations within the atherosclerotic lesions exhibit a high degree of correlation with the depth of the lesion in the artery wall, whereas Zn is observed to be anti-correlated to the size of the lesion area. This investigation implies that the observed high Fe levels, which can lead to increased free radical damage, may cause premature or accelerated arterial damage.[8]

Samples of healthy and carcinoma tissues from colon, breast, uterus in German population, and from the rectum, sigmoid, thyroid, kidney, larynx and lungs in Portuguese population were assessed for 30 TE, through TXRF and normal *Energy-dispersive X-ray fluorescence* (EDXRF). Results suggested an increased or constant levels of phosphor (P), sulfur(S), potassium (K), calcium (Ca), Fe and Cu, and decreased levels of Zn and bromine (Br) in carcinoma tissues. When comparing the results obtained for both techniques, the patterns were the same.[9]

Cerebro-spinal fluid (CSF)and blood levels of aluminum (Al), Cd, Ca, Cu, Pb, magnesium (Mg), and Hg were studied in seniors with dementia of the Alzheimer's type. Furthermore, As, Br, Cr, Fe, Mn, Ni, Rb, Se, Sr, and Zn were measured only in blood. The plasma levels of Al, Cd, Hg and Se were increased and the contents of Fe and Mn were lower in dementia. In cerebro-spinal fluid there were low levels of Cd and Ca, and increased content of Cu. Fe and Zn levels in blood and Ca in both blood and CSF correlated with memory and cognitive functions. Fe, Mn, and Sr levels in blood and Al in CSF were related with changes in behavior.[10]

In autism spectrum children, a statistically significant difference is found in the mean hair levels of As, Cd, Ba, Ce, Mg, Zn, and Pb compared to that from typically developing children. However, there are no statistically significant differences in the mean urine levels of Al, Ba, Ce, Hg, Cu, Pb, and germanium (Ge). In both, hair and urine specimens, agreement is found for barium (Ba) and Pb, only. [11]

When it comes to the counts of TE in biomedical samples from healthy or unhealthy individuals, the disparities between the reported values must be examined critically. There is solid experimental evidence that much of the existing controversy is due to inadequate sampling and sample handling, defective analysis, differences between blood, plasma, saliva, or spinal liquid TE-concentrations, or due to the limits of quantification of hardly traceable TE- concentrations.

In healthy and non-obese adults, the limits of quantification (LOQ) calculated to the undiluted blood range from 0.003 μg/L for uranium (U) to 0.1 μg/L for gallium (Ga). The geometric mean concentrations of nearly 37 TE in blood range from the LOQs in the lower ng/L-range up to 2369 μg/L for Rb. Essential TE concentrations in blood are in a small range for Mn (4.8-18 μg/L), Cu (720-1800 μg/L) and Se (85-182 μg/L). Other essential trace elements concentration ranges are 12-195 μg/L for boron (B), 0.04-0.8 μg/L for Co and 0.06-4 μg/L for Mo. Geometric mean concentrations of some toxic elements, such as Pb, Cd and Hg in blood are 19, 0,4 and 0,8 μg/L, respectively. For other toxic elements (Be, Th, U) or elements without a known biological function, such as hafnium (Hf), cerium (Ce), lanthanum (La), tellurium (Te) and gallium (Ga), many of the concentrations in the real samples are below the LOQs. [12]

The concentrations of Pb, Cd, Fe, Ni, Cu and Zn in the human semen in correlation to the occurrence of pathological spermatozoa were investigated with the help of the voltametric and flame absorption spectrophotometry methods. The concentrations in the semen were: Pb 1.49 mg x kg$^{(-1)}$, Cd 0.13 mg x kg$^{(-1)}$, Fe 2.59 mg x kg$^{(-1)}$, Ni 0.40 mg x kg$^{(-1)}$, Cu 0.28 mg x kg$^{(-1)}$, and Zn 153.93 mg x kg$^{(-1)}$. The total percentage of pathological spermatozoa was 41.6 % with predominance of broken flagellum, flagellum torso and separated flagellum. In relation to trace elements the analysis showed correlations between Cu and Pb (r = -0.47), Ni, Pb, Fe with flagellum ball (r = -0.39), Cd and large heads (r = 0.37). Findings suggest on possible effects of TE on the spermatozoa quality in normal human sperm.[13]

These findings are cross-validated by another study suggesting that the seminal plasma Zn concentration positively correlates with sperm concentration, sperm motility, and normal sperm morphology. [14]

The normal concentration of the essential TE in hair and saliva of normally developing healthy children aged 4-7 years are found to be: in hair - Fe 28.47mg/kg; Zn 172.1 mg/kg; Cu 21 mg/kg; Mn 1.3 mg/kg; in saliva- Fe 1.06 mg; Zn 0.64 mg; Cu 0.19mg; Mn 0.11 nmol/L. There is a correlation between Zn in saliva and hair ($P<0.05$). There is also a relatively low level of Mn in saliva compared with the proportion that meets the thresholds (0.11nmol/l) in children. The anthropometric data and socioeconomic status of children do not confound the levels of these elements in hair and saliva. The results indicate the possibility of assessing the presence of these elements using non-invasive methods in the absence of contamination and thus, they substantiate the potential of hair and saliva as a biomarker but could not ascertain the exact tolerable levels of TE in children.[15]

Erythrocyte levels of Se, Fe, Cu, Zn, Ca, and Mg are significantly higher and plasma levels of Cu, Ca, and Mg are significantly lower in patients with essential hyperhidrosis. [16]

The obtained data show that much work remains to be done to establish the normal levels of the most TE. The development of adequate measures for contamination control and the adjustments to the confounders (age, race, gender, body mass index, occupation, sleep patterns, parity, smoking) are the most important prerequisites.

ORGANIC FOOD VS. MINERAL SUPPLEMENTS

Our body is truly a masterpiece formed also from the trace elements in special, meaningful fabric and architecture. But it is important to understand, that constantly replenishing ourselves with the elements on a daily basis is an incorrect approach that does not work well.

Metabolic processes occurring in our body rely on the proper balance of trace minerals. Experts estimate 90 % of Americans suffer from mineral imbalance and deficiency. However, ingesting Fe, Ca, or Zn is not a supplementary solution to achieve that balance, because:

(1) Trace minerals do not exist by themselves, but in relationship to one another. Just ingesting some 60 elements in a pill is not what are body needs.

(2) Uncritical dosage of one TE (which is a possibility because of the trace amounts of the minerals) can lead to imbalances in others. For example the increase of Pb levels decreases Fe, the increase of the Cu levels decreases Zn, and the increase of Ca decreases Mg.

(3) Certain minerals are not digested in the intestine, as they require a favorable environment to be solved. For example, a Fe pill cannot be solved unless it is taken with an acidic liquid, such as vinegar, lemon juice, or ascorbic acid (Vitamin C).

(4) Most trace elements need to be in ionic form to be well absorbed in the small intestine. As food matter passes through the intestines, minerals transfer into the blood stream through the walls of the intestine by way of the

villi. This can only happen if the minerals are in an ionic form. Although stomach acid helps ionize the minerals in foods, a mineral supplement should contain already naturally ionized minerals to be fully absorbed.

(5) The overdose of any TE can be toxic and life threatening.

The excess in potassium (K) or *hyperkalemia,* is manifested in malaise, heart palpitations, muscle weakness, metabolic acidosis, renal insufficiency (from ineffective excretion), precancer, and even medical emergency or sudden death. Increased calcium (Ca) or hypercalcemia, results in renal or biliary stones, increased blood pressure, bone pain, nausea and vomiting, polyuria, pancreatitis, insomnia, depression, and coma.

Excessive zinc (Zn) (intake over 15 mg/day) leads to copper and iron deficiency, alters the metabolism of the cholesterol. There is also a condition called the "zinc shakes" or "zinc chills" or metal fume fever that can be induced by the inhalation of freshly formed zinc oxide. Typical levels of Zn in the plasma of healthy adults are 14 μmol L^{-1} (0.9 μg g^{-1}).

Copper (Cu) in the blood exist in two forms: bound to *ceruloplasmin* (85–95%) and the rest "free" loosely bound to *albumin* and small molecules. Free Cu causes toxicity, as it generates reactive oxygen species such as *superoxide, hydrogen peroxide,* and the *hydroxyl* radical. These damage proteins, lipids and DNA. Typical levels of Cu in the serum of healthy adults is 17 μmol L-1 (1.1 μg g^{-1}). Acute symptoms of *Cu poisoning* by ingestion include vomiting, hematemesis, hypotension, melena (black "tarry" feces), gastrointestinal distress, liver cirrhosis, Kayser-Fleischer rings (rings of Cu deposits in the cornea), jaundice, and coma.

The *iron (Fe) overload* is a disease called hemochromatosis. Hereditary hemochromatosis is an autosomal recessive disorder, characterized by an accelerated rate of intestinal Fe absorption and progressive Fe deposition. The most common presentation is hepatic cirrhosis in combination with hypopituitarism, cardiomyopathy, diabetes, arthritis, or hyperpigmentation.

The *manganese poisoning or manganism*, can lead to neuro-psychiatric symptoms, such as reduced response speed, irritability, mood changes, and compulsive behaviors, idiopathic Parkinson's disease, and multiple sclerosis.

Typical levels of Se in the serum of healthy adults are 2 µmol L-1 (0.16 µg g^{-1}). Symptoms of *excessive selenium or selenosis,* include a garlic odor on the breath, gastrointestinal disorders, hair loss, sloughing of nails, fatigue, irritability, and neurological damage. Extreme cases of selenosis can result in cirrhosis of the liver, pulmonary edema, cardio-respiratory arrest and death.

Symptoms of *excessive phosphorus or hyperphosphatemia* include ectopic calcification, secondary hyperparathyroidism, and renal osteodystrophy.

Acute cadmium poisoning may cause flu-like symptoms such as chills, fever, and muscle ache sometimes referred to as "the cadmium blues." Symptoms may resolve after a week if there is no respiratory damage. More severe exposures can cause tracheo-bronchitis, pneumonitis, and pulmonary edema. Ingestion of any significant amount of cadmium causes immediate poisoning and damage to the liver and the kidneys. Compounds containing cadmium are also carcinogenic. Other symptoms include anosmia (lose of the sense of smell), osteomalacia, osteoporosis, and spontaneous fractures. The kidney damage inflicted by cadmium poisoning is irreversible. The proximal renal tubular dysfunction creates hypophosphatemia, causing muscle weakness and sometimes coma. The dysfunction also causes gout, due to the hyperuricemia. Another side effect is hyperchloremia. The kidneys can also shrink up to 30%.

Eating fresh grains, fruits, vegetables grown in nutrient-rich organic soil is the primary and safest supply for a full spectrum of ionic minerals. An ion is a mineral or element that has a positive or negative charge. This unstable ionic state allows the element to bond readily with water, making it possible for the body to absorb it. Trace minerals exist plentifully and in proper proportions in the mineral-rich waters of the oceans and seas, for the TE abundant in soil are washed into the oceans. For example, in the Great Salt Lake of Utah or the Dead Sea in Israel, these essential elements exist in highly concentrated, salubrious proportions, eight to ten times more concentrated than regular seawater and even more dense than in sweet waters.

Today, trace minerals research offers over 100 different health promoting products. Nevertheless, promoting the organic meal culture (especially seafood and uncooked veggies and greens) is the most reliable method of sustaining the right mineral balance. Go for it!

HYPEREMESIS GRAVIDARUM

Hyperemesis gravidarum (HG) is a condition causing severe nausea and vomiting (10 times a day or more, without irritation) before the 22_{nd} weeks of pregnancy. The incidence of HG is approximately 0.3-2.3% of live births, and higher in multiple pregnancies, hydatidiform mole, and trophoblastic disease. Both the aetiology and pathogenesis of HG remain unknown, although concepts of defective placentation, autoimmune disturbances, genetic predisposition, infection (Helicobacter Pylori), thyroid dysfunction, low age, low body mass index prior to pregnancy, multiple pregnancies, are being discussed. Vomiting reflex can be also achieved through stumulation of trigeminus (V cranial nerve), glossopharyngeus (IX cranial nerve) and vagus (X cranial nerve). HG leads to anemia and severe dehyrdatation often resultant in hospitalization.

The *emetic reflex* (ER) is an autonomous defense reaction of the gastrointestinal tract, aimed at eliminating noxious agents in identical way as a cough or sneezing aimed at eliminating irritating particles from the respiratory passage. Nausea and emesis can also represent general symptoms of diseases or side effects of certain drug or physical actions (like chemotherapy or radiation).

The receptive pathway of the ER is a build-up of different sensors and receptors in the periphery as well as within the central neural system (CNS). Sensory impulses are conveyed by afferent neurons toward a medullary control center or so-called "vomiting center." In this center, impulses are integrated and transmitted onto motor and autonomic output to the digestive tract. The structures within the CNS that can be regarded as the central coordination areas of the ER, are presented in Figure 2:

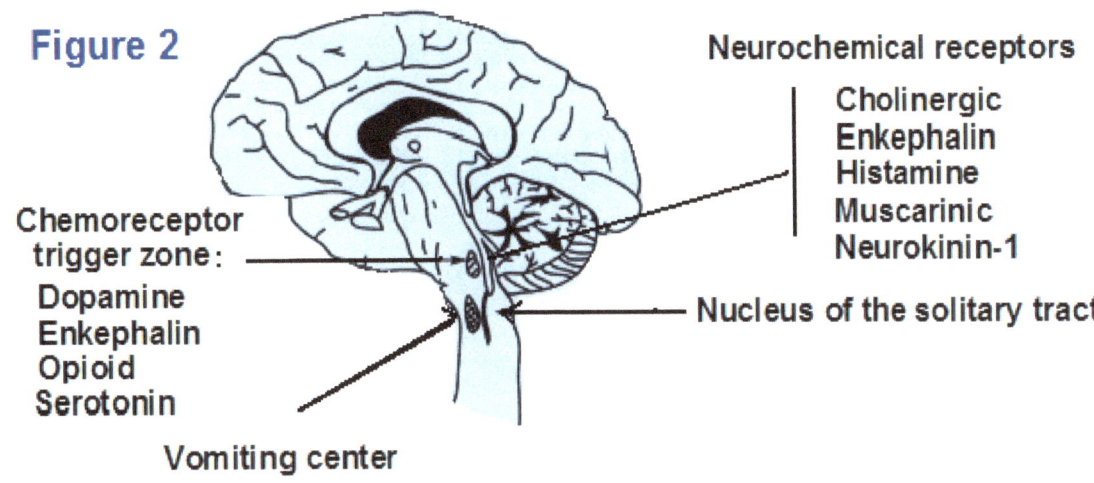

As shown in the figure, many neurotransmitter receptors are present on this reflex arc which can be selectively influenced by antiemetic drugs, hormones, and certain trace elements. Depending on the noxious agents and the anatomical location of the pathways, different receptors and factors are involved or effective.

Within the CNS there are three structures responsible for the ER coordination.[17] They are located in the medulla (brain stem). Vomiting is a subjective sensation, coordinated by a distributed medullary control system rather than a unique, well-defined vomiting center. Neurons involved are embedded in an arc of neurons radiating from the nucleus of the solitary tract (NST) through the intermediate reticular zone of the lateral tegmental field to the ventrolateral medulla. These functional areas are located close to the vagus nerve, the most important input for the ER.

The "chemoreceptor trigger zone" (CTZ) of the area postrema, is situated nearby, which serves the central detection of noxious agents that circulate in bloodstream and in the cerebrospinal fluid. This area seated on the floor of the 4th ventricle is on the one hand directly exposed to the cerebrospinal fluid and can detect noxious agents in it, and on the other hand it contains a dense vascular network of fenestrated capillaries. In this way, substances that do not penetrate the hemato-encephalic barrier, are detected in the bloodstream. Finally, chemoreceptors located outside the area postrema, are sensitive to circulating apomorphine, dopamine, oxidative stress, and cytotoxic drugs.

Due to increased metabolic requests, pregnancy can be considered as metabolic stress, especially if associated with oxidative stress triggered by disbalance of pro/antioxidants. Serum copper (Cu) and total serum antioxidant capacity (TAC) are significantly higher in hyperemesis gravidarum, while zinc (Zn) is lower in all pregnant groups regardless of hypertensive disorders. Iron (Fe) might have a role in etiopathogenesis of hyperemesis, while the increase of TAC in the very beginning of preeclampsia might represent a stress defense mechanism. [18]

Selenium (Se) deficiency is reported to be implicative in hyperemesis, obstetric cholestasis preeclampsia, fetal growth restriction, preterm labor, gestational diabetes. [19]

Another study has not shown significant changes in erythrocyte Zn, Cu and Mg concentrations in hyperemesis gravidarum. Plasma Zn levels however, are significantly higher, and plasma Cu levels are significantly lower. Treatment of hyperemesis brings a significant decrease in plasma Zn levels, and increase in plasma Cu concentration, but does not change the erythrocyte Zn, Cu, and Mg concentrations. Grouped according the degree of ketonuria, the levels of TE remain the same. [20]

These results are not supported by a study suggesting that there are no significant changes in serum Cu or Zn in patients with hyperemesis compared to normal pregnant women. Also, no significant correlations are found between the changes in the levels of these TE and the decrease in serum sodium (Na), potassium (K) and urinary chloride.[21]

Because the multilayer pathogenesis of the pernicious vomiting is not fully understood, and is attributed to hormones, gastrointestinal dysfunction, thyrotoxicosis, serotonin disbalance, hepatic abnormalities, autonomic nervous dysfunction, nutritional deficiencies, asthma, allergies, *Helicobacter pylori* infection, or psychosomatic causes, treatment of hyperemesis by replacement TE should be enacted very carefully.

Modification of the amount and size of daily meals rich carbohydrate in may help relieve symptoms. Protein-rich meals also decrease symptoms. Drinks that contain electrolytes and other supplements are advised. [22]

PREECLAMPSIA

Preeclampsia is a syndrome occurring in 6-8% of pregnancies and is characterized by the sequential development of edema, hypertension and proteinuria after the 20_{th} gestation weeks. Preeclampsia TE diagnosed when blood-pressure recordings in the lateral recumbent position or with a 15-30 degree tilt to the left side show a rise of systolic pressure that is greater than 30mm Hg or a rise of diastolic pressure that is greater than 15 mm Hg in two measurements of the both sides with 20 minute intervals, and in presence of proteinuria (protein concentration greater than 3 g/liter or 4+ on random sample).

The aetiology is unknown but the pathogenesis is found to be associated with systematic endothelial dysfunction in the capillary net, placental defects, increased placental mass, cardiovascular and renal diseases, coagulation diseases, uterine anomalies, among the others.

Preeclampsia is associated with oxidative stress in the maternal circulation. Decreased levels of Zn, Cu, Se, Mg, superoxide dismutase (SOD), glutathione peroxidase (GPx), and elevated levels of malondialdehyde (marker of lipid peroxidation) in the umbilical cord blood of preeclamptic pregnancies are observed. Positive correlations are found between Zn and antioxidant SOD (r = 0.581), as well as between Cu and SOD (r = 0.576), Se and antioxidant GPx (r = 0.445). The reduced levels of TE associated with inadequate amount of antioxidant enzymes may be important contributing factor leading to endothelial dysfunction in preeclampsia. [23]

A contradicting study suggests that Cu content of maternal serum and urine is increased in preeclamptic pregnancy.[24] Overall, increased Cu level, especially combined with low Zn, is a major concern in prognosis of preeclampsia, as the latter is associated with hypoproteinemia.

Increased oxidative stress due to endothelial dysfunction in preeclampsia is catalyzed in the presence of free transitional metals. Therefore, it is crucial to establish Fe and ferritin concentrations in maternal plasma of preeclamptic women. It is found, that mean serum Fe (23.48 µg/dL) and mean serum ferritin concentrations (32.56 µg/dL) are increased in preeclampsia in the absence of any differences in red blood cell indices, hemoglobin (Hb) concentration, hematocrit (Hct) compared to that from healthy pregnant women. [25]

Thus, plasma Fe is increased in preeclampsia when compared to healthy pregnant women. This is in contrast to inflammation characteristic for preeclampsia. The link between Fe homeostasis and inflammation is hepcidin. With the help of spectrophotometry it is found that plasma hepcidin, IL-6, Fe and ferritin concentrations are increased, whereas plasma transferrin, total iron binding capacity (TIBC), and mean corpuscular hemoglobin concentrations are lower in preeclampsia. [26]

In hypoxic newborns to mild preeclamptic mothers, the nonprotein-bound iron (NPBI) levels are decreased (1.86 micromol/L) in cord blood. [27]

Severe preeclampsia is associated with abnormal concentrations of Zn,

Cu, and Se. In patients with preeclampsia, Zn levels are found to be significantly higher in fetal arterial (947.3 µg/L) and venous blood (911.1 µg/L) samples. Se levels are significantly lower in maternal (98.6 µg/L) and fetal arterial (110.7µg/L) and venous cord blood (82 µg/L) samples. Cu levels are significantly lower in fetal arterial (581.6 µg/L) and venous cord blood (949 µg/L) samples, but higher in maternal blood (2264.6 µg/L). These differences remain significant while controlling for the mode of delivery. Interestingly, Mg levels are also higher in preeclampsia.[28]

Through a randomized, double-blind, placebo-controlled study it is established that Se supplementation in pregnant women may be associated with a lower frequency of preeclampsia. [29]

Urinary iodine excretion is seen to be the most convenient laboratory marker of iodine deficiency. Urinary iodine concentration might be a useful early marker in the assessment of preeclamptic women. The urinary iodine level (4.25 microg/dL) and blood magnesium concentration (1.63 mg/dL) are found to be decreased in Turkish women with severe preeclampsia with a positive correlation between urinary iodine and blood magnesium levels (Pearson coefficient = 0.43). It is concluded that iodine supplementation may be considered in the management of preeclampsia.[30]

Concentrations of Pb, Sb, Mn, Hg, Co, Zn in umbilical cord blood and mother whole blood were measured in 396 postpartum women without occupational exposure to metals in Iran, using inductively coupled plasma mass spectrometry. Preeclampsia was diagnosed in 7.8% of subjects. Levels of Pb, Sb and Mn in umbilical cord blood were significantly higher in preeclampsia (4.30 microg/dL, 4.16 microg/dL and 46.87 microg/L, respectively) . The logistic regression analysis revealed that one unit increase in the common logarithms of umbilical cord blood concentration of Pb, Sb or Mn led to increase in the risk of preeclampsia several-fold: unit risks were 12.96, 6.11, and 34.2 for Pb, Sb and Mn, respectively. These findings suggest that environmental exposure to Pb, Sb and Mn may increase the risk of preeclampsia in women without occupational exposure. [31]

Fairly different in their expressions, the above presented studies agree around one consistency: in preeclampsia, the levels of certain TE (Cu, Se, Zn) in maternal plasma are in negative correlations to that measured in fetal arterial and venous blood. Further research is essential to confirm this observation, that would help to better explain the pathogenesis of preeclampsia. It would help to understand whether the reciprocal levels of Cu or Zn in maternal and fetal plasma are related with placental absorption or metabolic alterations in pregnancy with preeclampsia. Correlated with further neonatal parameters, these findings would aid the therapy or prevention of the intrauterine growth retardation and prematurity.

GESTATIONAL DIABETES

Gestational diabetes (GD) is a condition in which women without previously diagnosed diabetes mellitus exhibit hyperglycemia and glycosuria during pregnancy (especially during the third trimester). It affects approximately 7% of all pregnancies (including the singleton and multiton). Diabetes mellitus is characterized by glucose intolerance and is closely related to TE. Investigation of changes of the trace elemental concentrations in plasma of the pregnant women with GD is significant for the treatment plan development.

An uneventful pregnancy even, favors oxidative stress because of the mitochondria-rich placenta. A transitional metal, especially Fe, which is particularly abundant in placenta, is important in the production of free radicals. Studies have shown that free Fe radicals have a role in GD. A case-control study has measured the Fe status, including ferritin, plasma Fe, total iron-binding capacity (TIBC), hemoglobin (Hb), mean corpuscular volume (MCV), and mean corpuscular hemoglobin (MCH). Concentration of serum ferritin, Fe, transferrin saturation and Hb, MCV, and MCH appear to be significantly higher, and TIBC significantly lower in GD. No significant association is observed with the familial history of diabetes and GD.[32]

Levels of Cu, Zn, Ca, Sr, Mg, P, Fe, and Al in the serum of pregnant women are determined and correlated with gestational weeks. The results show that compared with normal pregnant women, Cu contents in serum of pregnant women with GD are increased, and Zn contents are decreased. In addition, for all pregnant women, the Ca contents in serum have an obvious inverse correlation with gestational period.[33]

Micronutrient concentrations of Ni, Al, Cr, Mg, Fe, Zn, Cu, and Se are measured in serum of women with gestational diabetes between 24 and 28 weeks of gestation. There is no significant difference between the serum micronutrient level (Ni, Al, Cr, Mg, Zn, Cu, Se) in study and control groups except serum level of Fe which was significantly lower in GD.[34]

Cr has been shown to play a role in glucose intolerance, Type 2 diabetes mellitus, and GD. In addition, the diabetic neuropathy of a patient on parenteral nutrition are alleviated when supplemental Cr is added to total parenteral nutrition solutions. In a study conducted in China, supplemental Cr as Cr-picolinate has improved the blood glucose, insulin, cholesterol, and hemoglobin A1C in people with Type 2 DM in a dose dependent manner. Follow-up studies have confirmed the results. The requirement for Cr is related to the degree of glucose intolerance: 200 mg/day of supplemental Cr is adequate to improve glucose variables of those who are mildly glucose intolerant. However, people with more overt impairments in glucose tolerance and diabetes usually require more than 200 mg/day. The mechanism of action of Cr involves increased insulin binding, increased insulin receptor number, and increased insulin receptor phosphorylation. [35]

Another 2-year prospective gestational cohort study on 580 patients with GD has revealed no significant differences between the Cr levels in 2_{nd}

and 3_{rd} trimesters among the healthy and diabetic pregnant women. [36]

Zn and Cr deficiency are observed in Type 2 diabetics with an increase in Cu. In healthy pregnant subjects, T-cells and activated T-cells are increased in direct proportion to serum Mg and Se. In insulin-treated GD patients, T-cells are increased proportionally to serum Zn while in diet controlled GD cohort T-cells are correlated directly with serum Mg and Zn, and are correlated inversely with serum Cu. The results thus show a correlation between TE deficiency, increased lipid peroxidation and lymphocyte activation in GD. Dietary manipulation may point to improvement in existing approaches to management of GD. [37]

In animal studies boron (B) shows effects on triglycerides and glucose and may act as a metabolic regulator in several enzymatic systems. B levels and serum lipids (total cholesterol, high-density cholesterol, low density cholesterol, triglycerides, lipoprotein-A, apolipoprotein-A-I and apolipoprotein-B) are measured in maternal blood samples at 24-28 gestational weeks of women with mean age of 30 years. The median boron levels are 15.2 µg/L with no significant differences in GD and control groups. No correlation are found between lipids and B levels. Considering the evidence that B acts as a regulator of energy substrate utilization, the effect of dietary B on glucose metabolism deserves further research.[38]

Further research could afford a randomized double-blind design, compare TE levels in maternal and umbilical cord plasma, in correlations with the weight and adaptation counts of the newborns to mothers with GD.

PREMATURITY

Miscarriage is the spontaneous termination of a pregnancy at a stage where the embryo or fetus is incapable of surviving independently. Usually it is before the 22_{nd} week of pregnancy. When the fetus dies while in the uterus in $20-24_{th}$ weeks of pregnancy, the complication is termed a stillbirth. Preterm labor is the spontaneous termination of pregnancy with a live fetus between 23_{rd} and 73_{rd} weeks of gestation. Prematurity is the birth before the 37 weeks gestation, covering miscarriage, stillbirth, and preterm birth.

Low birth weight is defined by weight (regardless of gestational age); a weight of less than 2500 g constitutes low birth weight, and weight less than 1500 g is called *very low birth weight.*

Intrauterine growth retardation is defined as weight less than the 10th percentile for the gestational age at birth.

For example, an infant weighing 2600g at birth at 34 weeks gestation would be premature but would not have retarded growth. An infant weighing 1499 g at 31 weeks gestation would not be growth retarded but would be premature (or preterm) with very low birth weight.

Neonatal morbidity of prematurity is classified below:

I. *Pulmonary*

(1) Respiratory distress syndrome

(2) Bronchopulmonary dysplasia

(3) Pneumothorax and interstitial emphysema

II. *Cardiovascular*

(4) Hypotension

(5) Persistent fetal circulation

(6) Patent ductus arteriosus

(7) Sudden infant death syndrome

III. *Central nervous system*

(8) Intracranial hemorrhage

(9) Apnea/bradycardia

(10) Vision/hearing problems

IV. *Gastrointestinal*

(11) Necrotizing enterocolitis

(12) Inadequate nutritional

V. *Metabolic*

(13) Hypothermia

(14) Hypoglycemia

(15) Hypocalcemia

(16) Hypothyroid

(17) Jaundice

(18) Diabetes

VI. *Immunological*

(19) Rh conflict

(20) Lupus

(21) Glomerulonephritis

(22) Polycystic kidney disease

VII. *Infectious*

(23) Generalized sepsis

(24) Herpes simples, cytomegalovirus, rubella, toxoplasmosis gondii, chlamydia trachomatis, shigella, listeria monocytogenes, group B streptococcus, among others.

VIII. *Genital and urinary tract defects*

(25)   Hypospadia

(26)   Undescended testicle

(27)   Phimosis

(28)   Hydronephrosis

(29)   Renal agenesis

(30)   Prune belly syndrome

IX. *Psychosocial.*

It is established that copper (Cu) level increases and the selenium (Se) level decreases as an uneventful pregnancy advances.[39]

Maternal Se deficiency during early gestation is thought to be one of the factors responsible in the pathogenesis of spontaneous or recurrent miscarriages.[40] Se status has been studied regarding adverse pregnancy outcomes, with emphasis on those related to diminished antioxidant activity and increased oxidative stress. Studies report that Se plays an important role in neural tube defects, diaphragmatic hernia, premature birth, low birth weight, preeclampsia, glucose intolerance and gestational diabetes.[41]

Through randomized trials it has been established that the mean serum Se and hair Se concentrations of women who miscarried (42.8 ng/mL, 276 ng/g, respectively) are significantly lower than those of the control healthy mothers (50.2 ng/mL, 300 ng/g, respectively) and non-pregnant women (58.1 ng/mL, 315 ng/g, respectively). [42]

Low levels of zinc (Zn) and copper (Cu) are also associated with miscarriages. There are only a few reports regarding the fertility and outcome of pregnancy in Wilson's disease. Pregnancy does not seem to have adverse effect on the clinical course of Wilson's disease, but teratogenity is not seen with low-dose and zinc sulphate.[43]

Plasma Cu values in non-pregnant women range from 11.6-25.8 micromol/L. In healthy pregnant women, there is a constant trend of the increase of serum Cu. The mean serum Cu gives three significant peaks at the 22_{nd}, 27_{th} and 35_{th} gestational weeks. Serum Cu is much lower in miscarried pregnancies. [44]

Zn supplementation results in a small but significant reduction in preterm birth (risk ratio 0.86). [45] Concentrations of Zn, Co, bromine (Br,) rubidium (Rb) and gold (Au) were determined by neutron activation analysis (NAA) in maternal and umbilical cord blood serum. The concentrations of essential TE (Zn, Co) were significantly lower while levels of non-essential TE (Br, Rb) were similar or increased (Au) in serum of pregnant as compared to serum of non-pregnant women. The mean value of Zn in the umbilical cord was 1.9 times higher than that of mothers. However, no correlation existed between the Zn level in maternal and umbilical cord plasma. These data suggest that Zn is actively transported from mother to fetus through the placenta.[46]

$MgSO_4$ exposure before preterm birth is neuroprotective, reducing the risk of cerebral palsy and major motor dysfunction. Neonatal inflammatory cytokine levels correlate with neurologic outcome, leading us to assess the effect of $MgSO_4$ on cytokine production. Short-term exposure to a clinically effective $MgSO_4$ concentration in vitro substantially reduces the frequency of neonatal monocytes producing TNF-α and IL-6 under constitutive conditions, decreasing cytokine gene and protein expression, without influencing cell viability or phagocytic function. $MgSO_4$ reduces cytokine production in intrapartum women, term and preterm neonates, demonstrating effectiveness in those at risk for inflammation-associated adverse perinatal outcomes. [47]

Available evidence presents some limitations: most study designs do not allow conclusions about causal relationships; study populations, selection of subjects, research setting, procedures for defining sample size and analytical methods are often poorly described; many studies fail to adjust for important confounding variables. Population studies assessing the relationship between Se, Zn, Cu, Mg or Fe intake during pregnancy and health outcomes are scarce. Further research is still needed to clarify the role of TE in adverse pregnancy outcomes, especially those related to augmented oxidative stress.

ENDOMETRIOSIS

Endometriosis is the presence of extrauterine endometrial glands and stroma affecting 10% of women in reproductive age. Internal endometriosis or adenomyosis is when the abnormal endometrial lesions are found in endometrium and myometrium. External endometriosis is when these lesions appear and flourish outside the uterus: in fallopian tubes, on peritoneum, Villar's nodule, ovaries, vagina, cervix, vulva, bladder, in brain, lungs, kidneys, etc. The main symptoms are the cyclic pain and infertility.

Several mechanisms are proposed, but no single theory can satisfactorily account for the anatomic distribution of endometriosis:

(1) *Retrograde menstruation*- a theory that best explains the predominance of disease in the dependent portions of the pelvis and the high incidence in patients with menstrual outflow obstruction.

(2) *Celomic metaplasia*- this accounts for the rare finding of endometriosis in the pleural cavity. In addition, celomic metaplasia may be induced after irritation by menstrual debris from retrograde flow.

(3) *Lymphatic and hematogenous dissemination* - as endometriosis has been documented in the lymphatics and veins that drain uterus. This explains the distant endometriosis in umbilicus, lung, kidney, brain, or nasopharynx.

(4) *Immunological factors and angiogenesis* -play a key role. In women with

endometriosis, there is an alteration in the function of peritoneal macrophages, natural killer cells and lymphocytes, with production of growth factors and inflammatory mediators in the peritoneal fluid.[48]

It is suggested that oxidative stress secondary to elevated peritoneal fluid iron (Fe), or deficiency of peritoneal copper (Cu) might play a role in the development and progression of endometriosis. [49]

Several important endometriosis-specific genes overlap with those known to be regulated by Fe. Other genes are involved in oxidative stress. Fe has a significant impact on endometriotic-cell gene expression.[50]

It has been shown on animal models that the administration of 0,5 ml of 5 mM aqueous solution of dinitrosyl-iron complexes (DNIC) with cysteine alleviated the development of experimental endometriosis in rats induced by surgical way: the size of endometriosis decreased 1.85 times during 10 days. The effect was suggested to be due to cytotoxic action of nitrosonium molecules and ions (NO+) released from rapidly decomposed DNIC in on endometriotic tissues.[51]

The scarcity of studies on the role of Cu in endometriosis is alarming, for Cu has the account of being a pro-estrogen element. On the other hand, there are no empirical data about the role of Zn in treatment of endometriosis, for Zn is found to have pro-progesterone, immunomodulatory, anti-inflammatory and anti-oxidative effects.

PREMATURE OVARIAN FAILURE

Premature ovarian failure (POF) or premature ovarian insufficiency (POI) is the loss of function of the ovaries before age 40. A commonly cited triad for this condition is amenorrhea, hypergonadotropism, and hypoestrogenism.

The risk of POF increases in association with autoimmune aggression. Adequate intake of vitamin D and trace elements is required for the immune system to function efficiently.

Precise coordination of meiotic progression is a critical determinant of an oocyte's capacity to be fertilized successfully, and zinc (Zn) has emerged as a key regulatory element in this process. An early manifestation of a regulatory role for this transition metal is the significant increase in total intracellular Zn. This accumulation is essential for meiotic progression beyond telophase-I and the establishment of meiotic arrest at metaphase-II. The subsequent developmental event, fertilization, induces a rapid expulsion of labile Zn that is a hallmark event in meiotic resumption. Zn fluxes work, in part, by altering the activity of the cytostatic factor (CTSF), the cellular activity required for the establishment and maintenance of metaphase II arrest in the mature, unfertilized egg. Zn itself, is a central component of the CTSF. [52]

Women with POI have significantly higher serum copper (Cu) levels and copper-to-zinc (Cu/Zn) ratio but significantly lower serum vit D and Zn levels when compared with the healthy controls. Serum follicle-stimulating hormone levels are inversely correlated with Zn and vit D levels and positively correlated with the Cu/Zn ratio and Cu levels. Vit D levels are inversely correlated with follicle-stimulating hormone levels, Cu/Zn ratio, and Cu levels and positively correlated with Zn levels. [53]

Cigarette smoking is a lifestyle behavior associated with subfertility and POF. Cigarette smoke contains a number of chemicals, many of which are involved in the generation of reactive oxygen species, which can lead to apoptosis and autophagy. The relevance of autophagy to toxin-induced changes in ovarian function is largely unexplored. Exposure to cigarette smoke causes follicle loss, oxidative stress, activation of the autophagy pathway, and a decrease in manganese (Mn) superoxide dismutase expression, leading to autophagy-mediated follicle death.[54]

Hair-dressers constitute a major occupational group of female workers who are exposed to chemicals (B, Cd) that cause reproductive abnormalities (RR 1.90). The risk increases when adjusted and limited for the Caucasian women only (RR 3.24). [55]

Lead (Pb) and mercury (Hg) also contribute to the premature ovarian aging. [56]

It is wished that studies generate hypotheses for the replication of research in the possible mechanisms behind alterations in trace elements and vit D deficiency in women with POF and whether these changes could be used to screen for the risk of developing POF.

CERVICAL CANCER

Cervical cancer is a broad understanding. In order to better absorb the role of TE in pathogenesis, staging and treatment of the cervical cancer (CC), Table 1 below, presents the pathological classification of this cancer:

Table 1: Pathological classification and staging of cervical cancer

Adenocarcinoma of cervix	Glandular carcinoma or mucinous carcinoma of endocervix. (15% of cervical cancers)	World health Organization (WHO), National Cancer Institute (NCI)
Squamous cell carcinoma	Keratinizing carcinomas (well or moderately differentiated) composed of large cells, or non-keratinizing (poorly differentiated) carcinomas. (85% of cervical cancers)	WHO, NCI
Transformation zone	Area of squamous metaplasia that has replaced native columnar epithelium.	The International Federation of Gynecologists & Obstetricians (FIGO) [2000]
Squamocolumnar junction	Meeting of the squamous and columnar cells of the exocervix and endocervix, respectively	FIGO [2000]
Cervical intraepithelial neoplasia (CIN, dysplasia)	Cellular abnormalities that meet specific cytological features (chromatin clumping, increased nuclear/cytoplastic ratio, hyperchromatic nucleus, prominent nucleoli) for premalignant conditions.	FIGO [2000]
CIN 1, CIN-2, CIN-3	Epithelial thickness dictates whether lesions are designated as CIN I (mild), II (moderate), or III (severe) dysplasias.	FIGO [2000]
Carcinoma in situ (stage 0)	Non-invasive cancer that is confined to the layer of cells lining the cervix.	FIGO [2000] National Cancer Institute (NCU) [2001]
Stage I (A, A $_{1,2}$, B, B $_{1,2}$)	Cancer is spread into the connective tissue of the cervix but is confined to the uterus (3mm-4cm, or 0.13in - 1.6 in)	FIGO [2000]; NCI [2001]

Findings from the flame atomic absorption spectroscopy suggest that CC tissue contains significantly lower concentrations of Zn, Se, Ca; elevated Cu, Fe, and increased Cu/Zn ratio compared to that in non-lesion tissue. The serum levels of Zn, Se, Ca, Fe are found to be decreased, and Cu, Mn, Cu/Zn ratio increased in patients with CC. The 22.64 - fold increase of Cu, and the deficit of Zn (0.11), and Se (0.6), suggest on the alteration of Cu/Zn ratio in 90% of CC cases. [57] The serum Cu/Zn ratio is in linear correlation with the stage of the cancer and may be used as a valuable predictor. [58]

Another study investigates the relationship between TE and the incidence of CC. Quite similar to the previous study, it reveals that the tissue contents of Zn, Se, and Ca are lower, the Cu, Fe concentrations and Cu/Zn ratio are higher in CC tissue. There are no significant differences in the contents of six TE (Ca, Cu, Fe, Mn, Se, Zn) and Cu/Zn ratio between cervical myoma tissue and paired nonlesion tissue. Also, the Fe level and Cu/Zn ratio are significantly higher and the Zn, Se levels are lower in CC tissue than in myoma tissue. The serum Cu level and Cu/Zn ratio are higher in the CC group than the myoma group. After adjustment for age, occupation, life habit, and other covariates for the development of CC, the odds ratios are 22.64 for Cu, 0.11 for Zn, and 0.60 for Se. It is concluded, that the increased serum and tissue levels of Cu and the Zn and Se deficiency may be risk factors for the CC. [59]

It is wished that further studies evaluate stage-sensitive contents of TE in CC patients, adjusted for age, parity, smoking, and the HPV infection.

OVARIAN CANCER

Staging of any cancer is not only a prognostic tool, but also a mean of communicating and comparing treatment and outcomes between institutions. Staging also allows an evaluation of treatment plans that are used within one institution. Staging does not limit the treatment plan and therapy can be tailored to the characteristics of the malignancy in each patient.

Ovarian cancer is a cancerous growth derived of the ovary. Most (90%) ovarian cancers arise from the surface of the ovary. Surface epithelial-stromal tumor, also known as ovarian epithelial carcinoma, is the most common type of ovarian cancer. The fallopian tube could also be the source of some ovarian cancers. There is also a primary ovarian sarcoma, derived of the ovarian connective tissue, a rare malignancy with poor prognosis.

Table 2 presents the FIGO staging of primary carcinoma of ovary:

Table 2: FIGO staging of primary carcinoma of ovary	2-year survival (%)	5-year survival (%)
STAGE I **Growth limited to ovaries** ◆ **Ia:** One ovary, no ascites, capsule intact, no surface tumor ◆ **Ib:** Both ovaries, no ascites, capsule intact, no surface growth ◆ **Ic:** One or both ovaries with tumor on surface, capsule is ruptured, or ascites contain malignant cells or have positive peritoneal washings.	**80**	**70**

STAGE II **Growth on one or both ovaries with pelvic extension**
- **IIa:** Metastases to tubes and/or uterus.
- **IIb:** Metastases to other pelvic tissues.   **40**   **25**
- **IIc:** Tumor is either stage IIa or IIb with the addition of tumor on the surface of one or both ovaries, a ruptured capsule, or ascites with malignant cells or positive peritoneal washings.

STAGE III **Growth on one or both ovaries with extrapelvic metastasis, positive retroperitoneal nodes, or inguinal nodes or with metastases to liver surface, omentum, or small intestine.**
- **IIIa:** Tumor in true pelvis, negative nodes, and microscopic seedling on peritoneal surfaces.   **18**   **12**
- **IIIb:** Tumor on one or both ovaries with implants less than 2 cm on abdominal peritoneal surfaces; nodes are negative.
- **IIIc:** Abdominal implants greater than 2 cm diameter and/or positive peritoneal or inguinal nodes.

STAGE IV **Growth involving one or both ovaries with distant metastases. If pleural effusion is present, cytology must be positive. Liver parenchymal metastasis equals Stage IV.**   **5**   **0**

Analysis of variance, covariance, correlation coefficient, multiple correlation, and partial correlation coefficient statistical tests were applied to cesium (Cs), chromium (Cr), cobalt (Co), iron (Fe), rubidium (Rb), scandium (Sc), selenium (Se), and zinc (Zn) content in human ovaries in order to evaluate statistically the possible relationships between these trace elements at the ovary as an organ-unit, each ovarian phase separately, each morphological part independent of the ovarian phase, and between cortex and medulla within the ovarian phases. The element Cs seems to have a homogeneous distribution between cortex and medulla within reproductive and menopausal phase. Zinc shows a trend to have an antagonistic relation with Cs, Cr, Co, and Fe during fetal and reproductive phases and not during menopausal phase. The relationship between Zn and Cs when Fe is kept constant could be used as a tool for the decontamination of the ovary from an abnormal Cs content or for the inhibition of the accumulation of the same element to the ovarian tissue. [60]

Although zinc (Zn) and copper (Cu) concentrations in plasma and tissues of patients with ovarian carcinoma have extensively been studied, the precise role of these metals in carcinogenesis is not clearly understood.

Cu and calcium (Ca) concentrations in cancerous ovary samples are observed to be higher than those in noncancerous ovary tissues, whereas magnesium (Mg), iron (Fe), and Zn levels in cancerous ovary samples are the same as in noncancerous tissues. [61]

It is found that the effects of Zn in treatment of carcinoma ovary, are additive with cisplatin or doxorubicin, whose morphological effects are distinct from those of Zn. Cytotoxicity of paclitaxel is minimal, making it difficult to determine additivity with Zn. Paclitaxel results in changes in cell shape and size similar to those of Zn but has different effects on cell cycle progression and cyclic expression. The data indicate that the means by which zinc kills ovarian cancer cells is distinct from currently used chemotherapeutics. Zn has the potential to be developed as either a primary treatment or as a second line of defense against cancers that have developed resistance to currently used chemotherapeutics.[62]

INDEX OF TERMS

Total reflection X-ray fluorescence analysis	TXRF	*3, 10, 46*
Total serum antioxidant capacity	TAC	*20*
Trace elements	TE	*3, 4, 6, 7-15, 17, 19, 21, 22, 25, 26, 28, 33, 37-39, 40, 42, 45-50*
Uranium	U	*12*
Visible/near infrared atomic absorption spectroscopy	Vis/NIR	*3*
World Health Organization	WHO	*39*
Zinc	Zn	*3,6, 10-15, 20-28, 32-38, 40, 42, 43, 45, 47, 49, 50*

REFERENCES:

1) **Shao Y, He Y (2013).**Visible/Near infrared spectroscopy and chemometrics for the prediction of trace element (Fe and Zn) levels in rice leaf. *Sensors (Basel); 13(2):1872-83*

2) **Nelson S, Barrows J, Haftmann R et al (2013).**Calculating the refractive index for pediatric parenteral nutrient solutions. American *Journal of Stem Pharmac; 70(4):350-5*

3) **Rogul'skiĭ IuV, Danil'chenko SN, Lushpa AP, Sukhodub LF (1997).** Measurement of trace elements in blood serum by atomic absorption spectroscopy with electrothermal atomization. *Klin Lab Diagn; (9)24:33*

4) **Wolf RE (2005).** What is ICP-MS, and more importantly, what can it do? Crustal Geophysics and Geochemistry Science Center. *Report Article.*

5) **Application Note (AN_E0649).** X Series ICP-MS Clinical Applications Note 5: Trace element quantification in blood and serum in a single analytical *run. Thermo.com*

6) **Lee FF (2007).** Comprehensive analysis, Henry's law constant determination, and photocatalytic degradation of polychlorinated biphenyls (PCBs) and/or other persistent organic pollutants. Ph. D. *dissertation, State University of New York at Albany, pp. 199-201*

7) **von Czarnowski, D.; Denkhaus, E.; Lemke, K (1997).** Determination of trace element distribution in cancerous and normal human tissues by total reflection X-ray fluorescence analysis. *Spectroscopy; 52 (7): 1047-1052*

8) **Minqin R, Watt F, Tan KH et al (2003).** Trace elemental distributions in induced atherosclerotic lesions using nuclear microscopy. *Nuclear Instruments and Methods in Physics Research Section B: Beam Interactions with Materials and Atoms; 210: 336-342*

9) **Magalhães T, von Bohlen A, Carvalho ML, Becker M (2006).**Trace elements in human cancerous and healthy tissues from the same individual: A comparative study by TXRF and EDXRF. *Spectrochimica Acta Part B: Atomic Spectroscopy; 61 (10-11):1185-1193*

10) **Basun H, Forssell LG, Wetterberg L, Winblad B (1991).** Metals and trace elements in plasma and cerebrospinal fluid in normal aging and Alzheimer's disease. *Journal of Neural Transmission in Parkins Dis and Dementia; 3(4):231-58*

11) **Blaurock-Busch E, Amin OR, Rabah T (2011).** Heavy metals and trace elements in hair and urine of a sample of Arab children with autistic spectrum disorder. *Maedica; 6(4): 247–257*

12) **Heitland P, Köster H (2006).** Biomonitoring of 37 Trace Elements in Human Blood and Plasma From Inhabitants of Northern Germany By ICP-MS. *Epidemiology; 17 (6): S299*

13) **Slivkova J, Popelkova M, Massanyi P et al (2009).** Concentration of trace elements in human semen and relation to spermatozoa quality. *Journal of Environmental Science Health A Tox Hazard Subst Env Eng; 44(4):370-5*

14) **Vickram S, Muthugadhalli S, Jayaraman G et al ().** Influence of trace elements and their correlation with semen quality in fertile and infertile subjects. *Gene Cloning Technology Lab, School of Biosciences and Technology, VIT University, Vellore, India*

15) **Ogboko B. (2011).** Trace element indices in hair and saliva of school children. J. *Basic. Appl. Sci. Res; 1(3):169-177*

16) **Güder H, Karaca S, Cemek M et al (2011).** Evaluation of trace elements, calcium, and magnesium levels in the plasma and erythrocytes of patients with essential hyperhidrosis. *International Journal of Dermatology; 50(9):1071-4*

17) **Donnerer J (2003).** Antiemetic therapy. *Karger Publisher; Switzerland* (Paperback).

18) **Fenzl V, Flegar-Meštrić Z, Perkov S et al (2013).** Trace elements and oxidative stress in hypertensive disorders of pregnancy. *Archives of Gynecology and Obstetrics; 287(1):19-24*

19) **Mistry HD, Broughton Pipkin F et al (2012).** Selenium in reproductive health. *American Journal of Obstetrics and Gynecology; 206(1):21-30*

20) **Dökmeci F, Engin-Ustün Y, Ustün Y et al (2004).** Trace element status in plasma and erythrocytes in hyperemesis gravidarum. *Journal of Reproductive Medicine; 49(3):200-4*

21) **el Tabbakh G, Darwish E, el Sebaie F et al (1989).** Study of serum copper and zinc in cases of hyperemesis gravidarum. *International Journal of Gynecology and Obstetrics; 29(3):207-13*

22) **Wegrzyniak LJ, Repke JT, Ural SU (2012).** Treatment of hyperemesis gravidarum. *Rev Obstetrics and Gynecology; 5(2): 78–84*

23) **Negi R, Pande D, Karki K et al (2012).** Trace elements and antioxidant enzymes associated with oxidative stress in the pre-eclamptic/eclamptic mothers during fetal circulation. *Clinical Nutrition; 31(6):946-50*

24) **Ranjkesh F, Jaliseh HK, Abutorabi S (2011).** Monitoring the copper content of serum and urine in pregnancies complicated by preeclampsia. *Biol Trace Elem Res; 144(1-3):58-62*

25) **Siddiqui IA, Jaleel A, Kadri HM et al (2011).** Iron status parameters in

preeclamptic women. *Archives of Gynecology and Obstetrics; 284(3):587-91*

26) **Toldi G, Stenczer B, Molvarec A et al (2010).** Hepcidin concentrations and iron homeostasis in preeclampsia. *Clin Chem Lab Med; 48(10):1423-6*

27) **Karadeniz L, Coban A, Ince Z et al (2010).** Cord blood cardiac troponin T and nonprotein-bound iron levels in newborns of mild pre-eclamptic mothers. *Neonatology; 97(4):305-10*

28) **Katz O, Paz-Tal O, Lazer T et al (2012).** Severe pre-eclampsia is associated with abnormal trace elements concentrations in maternal and fetal blood. *Journal of Maternal Fetal and Neonatal Medicine; 25(7):1127-30*

29) **Tara F, Maamouri G, Rayman MP et al (2010).** Selenium supplementation and the incidence of preeclampsia in pregnant Iranian women: a randomized, double-blind, placebo-controlled pilot trial. *Taiwan Journal of Obstetr Gynecol; 49(2):181-7*

30) **Gulaboglu M, Borekci B, Delibas I (2010).** Urine iodine levels in preeclamptic and normal pregnant women. *Biol Trace Elem Res; 136(3):249-57*

31) **Vigeh M, Yokoyama K, Ramezanzadeh F et al (2006).** Lead and other trace metals in preeclampsia: a case-control study in Tehran, Iran. *Environmental Research; 100(2):268-75*

32) **Afkhami-Ardekani M, Rashidi M (2009).** Iron status in women with and without gestational diabetes mellitus. *Journal of Diabetes Complications; 23(3):194-8*

33) **Wang Y, Tan M, Huang Z et al (2002).** Elemental contents in serum of pregnant women with gestational diabetes mellitus. *Biol Trace Elem Research; 88(2):113-8*

34) **Akhlaghi F, Bagheri SM, Rajabi O (2012).** A comparative study of relationship between micronutrients and gestational diabetes. *Obstetrics and Gynecology; Article ID 470419*

35) **Anderson RA (1998).** Chromium, glucose intolerance and diabetes. *Journal of the American College of Nutrition; 17(6): 548–555*

36) **Woods SE, Ghodsi V, Engel A et al (2008).** Serum chromium and gestational diabetes. *Journal of the American Board of Fam. Med; 21(2):153-7*

37) **Mahmoud F, Abul H, Dashti A et al (2012).** Trace elements and cell-mediated immunity in gestational and pre-gestational diabetes mellitus at third trimester of pregnancy. *Acta Med Acad; 41(2):175-85*

38) **Caglar GS, Cakal GO, Yüce E, Pabuccu R (2011).** Evaluation of serum boron levels and lipid profile in pregnancies with or without gestational diabetes. *Perinatal Medicine; 40(2):137-40*

39) **Nwagha UI, Ogbodo SO, Nwogu-Ikojo EE et al (2011).** Copper and selenium

status of healthy pregnant women in Enugu, southeastern Nigeria. *Niger J Clin Practice; 14(4):408-12*

40) **Mistry HD, Broughton PF, Redman CW, Poston L (2012).** Selenium in reproductive health. *American Journal of Obstet and Gynecol; 206(1):21-30*

41) **Mariath AB, Bergamaschi DP, Rondó PH et al (2011).** The possible role of selenium status in adverse pregnancy outcomes. *Br J of Nutrition; 105(10):1418-28*

42) **Müzehher G, Hüseyin G, Fikret K et al (2002).** Low levels of selenium in miscarriage. *The Journal of Trace Elements in Experimental Medicine; 15 (2):97-101*

43) **Sinha S, Taly AB, Prashanth LK et al (2004).** Successful pregnancies and abortions in symptomatic and asymptomatic Wilson's disease. *Journal of Neurolog. Sci; 217(1):37-40*

44) **Vukelić J, Kapamadzija A, Petrović D et al (2012).** Variations of serum copper values in pregnancy. *Srp Arch Celok lek; 140(1-2):42-6*

45) **Mori R, Ota E, Middleton P et al (2012).** Zinc supplementation for improving pregnancy and infant outcome. *Cochrane Database of Syst Rev; 7:CD000230*

46) **Alexiou D, Grimanis AP, Grimani M et al (1970).** Concentrations of zinc, cobalt, bromine, rubidium and gold in maternal and cord blood serum. *Neonatology; 28(3-4):191-195*

47) **Sugimoto J, Romani AM, Valentin-Torres AM et al (2012).** Magnesium decreases inflammatory cytokine production: a novel innate immunomodulatory mechanism. *Journal of Immunology; 188(12):6338-46*

48) **Larosa M, Facchini F, Pozzoli G et al (2010).** Endometriosis: aetiopathogenetic basis. *Urologia; 77 Suppl 17:1-11*

49) **Osman HG, El-Refaey AA, El-Sokkary AM, El-Saeed RA (2012).** Role of some trace elements in the physiopathology of endometriosis. *Journal of Endometriosis; 4(2): 68 - 76*

50) **Kobayashi H, Yamada Y, Kanayama S et al (2009).** The role of iron in the pathogenesis of endometriosis. *Gynecological Oncology; 25(1):39-52*

51) **Burgova EN, Tkachev NA, Vanin AF (2012).** The dinitrosyl-iron complexes with cysteine block the development of experimental endometriosis in rats. *Biofizika; 57(1):105-9*

52) **Bernhardt ML, Kong BY, Kim AM et al (2012).** A zinc-dependent mechanism regulates meiotic progression in mammalian oocytes. *Biol Reprod; 86(4):114*

53) **Kebapcilar AG, Kulaksizoglu M, Kebapcilar L et al (2013).** Is there a link between premature ovarian failure and serum concentrations of vitamin D, zinc, and copper? *Menopause; 20(1):94-9*

54) **Gannon AM, Stämpfli MR, Foster WG (2013).** Cigarette smoke exposure elicits increased autophagy and dysregulation of mitochondrial dynamics in murine granulosa cells. *Biol Reprod; Jan 16. [Epub ahead of print]*

55) **Gallicchio L, Miller S, Greene T et al. (2009).** Premature ovarian failure among hairdressers. *Human Reproduction; 24(10): 2636-2641.*

56) **Swanton A, Child T(2005).** Reproduction and ovarian aging. *Menopause International; 11(4):126-131.*

57. **Chan CA, Hwang JL, Kuo TL et al (1990).** Serum copper and zinc levels in patients with cervical cancer. *Journal of the Formosan Medical Association; 89(8):677-82*

58. **Brandes JM, Lightman A, Drugan A et al (1983).** The diagnostic value of serum copper/zinc ratio in gynecological tumors. *Acta Obstetrica et Gynecologica Scandinavica; 62(3):225-9.*

59. **Cunzhi H, Jiexian J, Xianwen Z et al (2003).** Serum and tissue levels of six trace elements and copper/zinc ratio in patients with cervical cancer and uterine myoma. *Biologic Trace Element Research; 94 (2): 113-122*

60. **Kania GD, Kouri E (1996).** Biological evaluation of trace element data in human ovaries by statistical analysis. *Biol Trace El Research; 52(1):65-116*

61. **Yaman M, Kaya G, Simsek M (2007).** Comparison of trace element concentrations in cancerous and noncancerous human endometrial and ovary tissues. *International J of Gynec Cancer, Official J of the International Gynecological Cancer Society; 17(1):220-228*

62. **Bastow M, Kriedt CL, Baldassare J et al (2011).** Zinc is a potential therapeutic for chemoresistant ovarian cancer. *J Exp Ther Oncol; 9(3):175-81*